HOW TO DO INTERMITTENT FASTING:
COMEPLETE GUIDE

DR.N.THOMAS

Disclaimer

All the material contained in this book is provided for educational and informational purposes only. No responsibility can be taken for any results or outcomes resulting from the use of this material.

While every attempt has been made to provide information that is both accurate and effective, the author does not assume any responsibility for the accuracy or use/misuse of this information.

You are encouraged to print this book for easy reading.

Use this information at your own risk.

Contents

INTRODUCTION

There is no denying it. Obesity has reached epidemic proportions and is prevalent in most of the Western nations. In fact, it is starting to spread to Asia too and people are increasingly becoming overweight and obese.

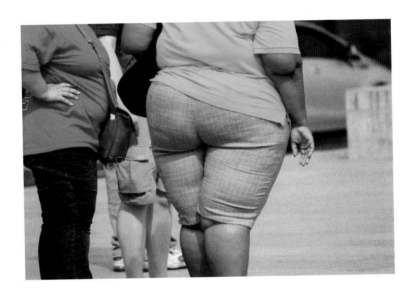

So, why is this happening? Why are there more overweight people now than ever before?

There are a few reasons for this. The first reason is our diet. Far too many people are addicted to junk food, processed food, white flour products, etc.

All these foods cause blood sugar levels to spike and this in turn leads to fat storage and insulin insensitivity.

A sedentary lifestyle is the second reason. With the advent of technology, many manual tasks have become easier and less demanding.

Need to go to the supermarket that's a 20 minute walk away?

Get the car instead of walking.

Need to go up to level 3 in your office building?

Take the elevator instead of the stairs.

All these activities that burn calories are avoided and replaced with easier alternatives. As a result, people are much more prone to gaining weight.

It's so much simpler to watch TV with a bag of potato chips than to go for a run. It's so much easier to drink a bottle of processed apple juice than eating a raw apple.

It's all these little actions that matter.

To exacerbate the situation, in the US, junk food is often cheaper than healthy, nutritious food. Low income families are able to easily purchase junk food but struggle to pay for "real food". This is one reason why obesity affects the low income families much more.

There is one cure to reversing weight gain and obesity. In fact, it is so powerful that people are able to lose weight even on a junk food diet just by adopting this method.

It is called intermittent fasting. We'll refer to it as **IF** from now on to make things easier. Unlike diets such as the Atkins diet or lemonade diet, intermittent fasting is a very unique method that doesn't concern itself with the food consumed. It is more focused on meal timings.

If you're struggling to lose weight or if you have an appetite that you can't control, intermittent fasting is your answer.

If you are trying to see your abs but just can't burn off the last layer of fat on your belly, intermittent fasting has your name written all over it.

This is truly one of the most effective and remarkable methods of losing weight.

Read on...

CHAPTER 1 – WHAT IS INTERMITTENT FASTING?

Intermittent fasting, just like its name suggests, is a cyclical diet that involves a period of fasting followed by a period of nonfasting. The non-fasting period may vary depending on the type of intermittent fasting you engage in.

There are several types of intermittent fasting. This report will highlight a few of the popular ones and recommend the easiest type to follow to ensure that your life does not become miserable.

The intermittent fasting can be broken down into 2 "windows".

- Fasting window
- Eating window

During the fasting window, you will not be allowed to consume any food. You can only drink water. No calories should be consumed during the fasting window.

During the eating window, you will be allowed to eat and will need to consume all your calories for the day during this window.

Intermittent fasting does not concern itself with what you eat. The diet is secondary. What really matters is that you MUST be compliant during the fasting period. This is when the body will utilize its fat stores for energy.

The principle of fasting is that when your stomach is empty, the body will not have food for fuel and will tap into its fat stores for fuel. This is imperative in burning fat successfully.

Many people struggle to lose weight because their insulin stores are full and the body burns food as fuel. The body never gets a chance to access the fat stores. As a result, even with exercise, the visible changes are slow to come.

It must be noted that even if you've adopted intermittent fasting, you should strive to be on a caloric deficit to guarantee fat loss. You can find out what your calorie requirements are by visiting http://www.freedieting.com/tools/calorie_calculator.htm

When you are at a caloric deficit and you combine it with intermittent fasting, your fat is going to melt off faster than what you ever thought possible.

Let's look at an example. If you have an 8-hour eating window and a 16 hour fasting window, you will need to consume all your calories for the day during the 8 hours.

The beauty about IF is that your body will not go into "starvation mode" because you will be eating and consuming calories. You're just doing it within a short span of time.

So, assuming you consume all your calories during the 8 hours, about 3 to 4 hours after your last meal, the food you ate would have been digested and some may have been used as fuel by your body.

However, there are about 12 hours left to go before your next meal since you're on a 16 hour fast. Your body will not have any more food to use as fuel.

That is when it will use the insulin and fat stores for energy. It doesn't matter if you're awake or sleeping; your body will still be burning calories for all the different bodily processes such as repair and maintenance. These calories will be coming from your stored fats.

This is what makes IF so fantastic. Like Leonardo da Vinci said, "Simplicity is the ultimate sophistication".

Intermittent fasting is extremely simple in concept. It doesn't involve detoxification, low carbs, ketogenic dieting, etc. None of that is an issue.

All you need to do is eat and fast... that's it. It doesn't get any simpler. *Now let's look at how it came about...*

CHAPTER 2 – COMMON QUESTIONS ABOUT INTERMITTENT FASTING

Where Did It Originate From?

There is no one particular place where IF originated from. In fact, it is based upon the way our ancestors ate.

In the past, food was scarce. If you wanted to eat, you had to hunt. On days when you managed to forage for food or the hunt was successful, there'd be a feast.

If the pickings were slim and there was no food, you'd go hungry. This would be akin to fasting. The only difference is that there wasn't a choice in the past.

Because of this manner of eating and fasting, our ancestors were seldom overweight. They also led much more active lives since there was no technology to assist them.

So, we can assume to certain degree that the human body instinctively adapts to intermittent fasting. We may have evolved technologically. However, when it comes to our physiology, we're pretty much the same as our ancestors.

Is Intermittent Fasting Safe for Me?

It depends. Nothing is perfect for everybody and this applies to IF too.

For most people, intermittent fasting will be safe. In fact, it will be highly beneficial. Studies have shown that many people who started an intermittent fasting program experienced health benefits such as increased fat burning and a higher metabolic rate.

Their blood pressure, bad cholesterol levels, blood sugar levels improved dramatically.

If you worry about intermittent fasting, you should allay your fears. Everybody goes through a fasting period when they are asleep. If you sleep for 8 hours, you will be in a fasted state.

The reason that many people do not enjoy the benefits of this fasted state is due to the fact that most people get less than 8 hours of sleep. Furthermore, people eat before bed. So, when they are sleeping, the food is being digested. The body doesn't get a chance to be in a fasted state for too long.

The moment they wake up, they have breakfast and start eating throughout the day. There is very little time for the body to tap into its fat stores.

People with gastric problems, diabetes, etc. should consult a doctor before starting an intermittent fasting program. Your doctor will be the best person to advise you if you should fast intermittently.

CHAPTER 3 – WHICH TYPE OF IF SHOULD YOU ADOPT?

There are several different types of intermittent fasting. Usually, the differences will depend on the person creating the method. The fundamentals of an eating window and a fasting window will ALWAYS apply.

Bear in mind that it really doesn't matter which method you choose. All the different methods will reap rewards. You should pick one that you're comfortable with.

When the method you choose is easy for you to follow, the chances of you complying with it and staying the course will be much higher. Initially, if you're new to intermittent fasting, you will want to take it slow and have a longer eating window and a shorter fasting window.

It will take about 2 weeks to a month for your body to adapt to your new way of eating. There is no doubt that you will most probably encounter resistance and cravings from your body.

This is par for the course. After all, most people are used to eating throughout their waking hours. Restricting your eating hours can be stressful in the beginning.

Rest assured that with time, your body will adapt and you will be surprised to see that your appetite has decreased. You will also feel more alert, energetic and slimmer as you progress.

Now let's look at some of the intermittent fasting methods.

Intermittent Fasting Method 1

The first one was created by Martin Berkhan of LeanGains.com. In fact, his method of IF is the most popular one out there. It is highly effective and relatively easy to follow.

The rules are that men will fast for 16 hours and women for 14 hours. They will have an 8 hour and 10 hour eating window respectively.

It is of paramount importance to keep your feeding window consistent. Failure to do so will confuse your body and impede your results.

Martin recommends scheduling your meals around your workouts. For example, if your feeding window ends at 7 pm, you should work out around 5.30pm and consume and complete your meal just before 7pm. Or you could start your eating window just after your workout. In this way, your body will have food to repair your muscles, etc.

Intermittent Fasting Method 2

The second method is known as the Warrior Diet and was created by Ori Hofmekeler.

This is a much more severe method that Martin's one. The rules state that you'll need to fast for 20 hours a day and only eat 1 large meal every night. This is supposedly what our ancestors may have done.

While it's anyone's guess as to whether our ancestors really ate in this manner, the fact remains that Ori's method is highly effective.

Many people who adopted his method have seen vast benefits to their health.

Initially when you're starting out, you might not want to use Ori's method. It would be a better idea to start off with Marin's method and gradually reduce your eating window over time till you are able to fast for 20 hours without discomfort.

Don't jump into the deep end of the pool and struggle with a 20 hour fast. You should also know that Ori's method does allow a few small meals during the fasting window. However, there are rules as to what you can eat and cannot eat.

So, you will need to watch your diet and stick to the approved food list. This is definitely one of the stricter methods of IF.

Intermittent Fasting Method 3

The third method of intermittent fasting is known as Eat Stop Eat and was created by Brad Pilon. His program is actually an online bestseller.

The rules of the fast are pretty simple. You will fast for 24 hours twice or thrice a week. On days when you're not fasting, you may eat what you want without worry.

In this manner, your overall consumption of calories for the week will be less and you will lose weight. Since you are allowed to eat whatever you want to eat during the eating window, you will not be deprived of your favorite foods.

This can be a relief to many people who fear giving up the foods they love. However, the 24 hour break from eating can be extremely difficult for many people. So, as mentioned earlier, you may follow Martin's method and work your way up.

How do you decide?

The truth of the matter is that you should analyze your eating habits, your sleeping patterns, your job requirements, etc. You MUST tailor the fast to suit you.

If you work nights, you can't fast through the night because you will be hungry. So, you should include your sleeping hours into your fasting window and maybe start your eating window 6 hours after waking.

Of course, this is assuming that you adopt the first type of intermittent fasting. You may also have social activities, etc. that may make following the intermittent fasting program difficult.

Sooner or later, your fasting will cramp your social life. Once again, you will need to work around it. Even the actor, Hugh Jackman, was on an intermittent fasting program while training for his Wolverine movie and he had to ensure that he stuck to his eating window despite his hectic schedule.

Ultimately, you must choose a method that you think will work for you. Do not get over-ambitious or overestimate your willpower and choose to go for the 24 hour fast on the first day.

It can and most probably will be torturous. You might end up giving up and eating. Later on, you may experience feelings of guilt and may feel like you failed. This is where most people throw in the towel.

They think they have failed when in reality, they just set unreasonable goals. The key to success is to make measurable progress with reasonable goals.

"Inch by inch, life's a cinch. Yard by yard, life is hard."

CHAPTER 4 – SHOULD YOU WATCH YOUR DIET?

Definitely. Regardless if you're on the intermittent fasting program or not, you should always pay close attention to what you're eating.

The number one cause of obesity and health problems is the food we eat. The truth of the matter is that deep down in our hearts, we know what we should be eating.

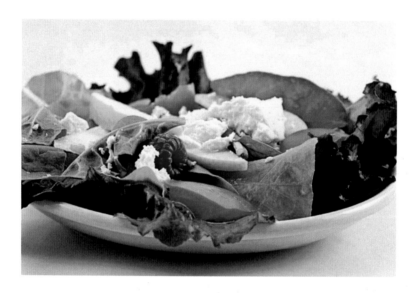

Vegetables and fruit are crucial to good health. They are packed with vitamins, minerals, antioxidants and fiber. The human body craves for vegetables.

However, our current diet is more focused on processed meats and there is just a cursory serving of vegetables that in most cases, does more damage than good.

French fries, hash browns and mashed potatoes in gravy sauce are not vegetables. You want to be consuming vegetables such as broccoli, kale, celery, tomatoes, cabbages, cucumbers, etc.

It is true that these vegetables may be more bland than the French fries. However, they are immensely beneficial to your health. Getting into the habit of eating vegetables will serve you well in the long run.

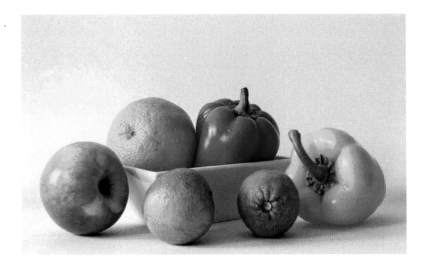

Vegetables are especially important during intermittent fasting. You can eat much more vegetables and still maintain your calorie count because vegetables generally contain fewer calories.

Furthermore, they will be more filling and you will be less likely to feel hunger pangs during the fasting window.

The same applies for fruit. Consume a wide variety of fruit and make sure they are 100% natural. Always eat the fruit rather than just drinking the juice. The fiber will do your body good and your insulin levels will be stable.

Avoid processed fruit that come in cans. Commercially sold juices should also be avoided because they are full of additives and sugar. Both are detrimental to your health.

Besides vegetables, you should get your proteins from healthy cuts of meat.

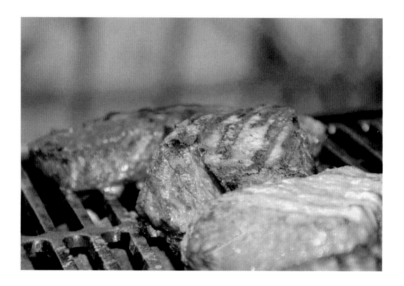

Prepare your meats in a healthy manner either by grilling them or steaming them. You may lightly sauté your meats if you prefer.

Deep fried meats and processed meats such as sausages and spam should be avoided or consumed minimally. They are highly fattening and contain a lot of calories and additives.

Besides proteins from meat and carbs from vegetables, you will also need healthy fats. There are 2 excellent sources of healthy fats; extra virgin olive oil and virgin coconut oil.

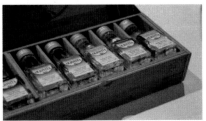 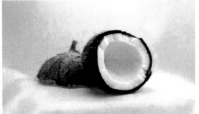

Out of the two oils, coconut oil is the superior one. The olive oil industry has been infiltrated by the Italian mafia and most of the commercially sold olive oils have been diluted and compromised.

Coconut oil is still untouched and extremely beneficial. In the past, it used to have a bad reputation for causing high levels of cholesterol, etc. However, latest studies have shown that this is false and coconut oil is actually very beneficial for one's health.

Since this guide is about intermittent fasting, we'll not be going into too much detail about diet and nutrition because there is so much to learn. You should do your own research on nutrition and clean eating so that you are better informed.

Intermittent fasting is so powerful that even if you ate junk food but maintained your caloric deficit, you would still lose weight.

However, your goal should be to lose weight and be healthy.

Losing weight is not the be all and end all. The best way to be healthy is to eat healthy. All the exercise in the world will not make you healthy if your diet is poor.

You may be lean and fit… but if the foods you eat are unhealthy, you will encounter health problems sooner or later. Go online and research what beneficial foods you should be eating and what health benefits are accrued from the consumption of these foods..

Gradually eliminate your bad food choices and replace them with healthier choices. For example, replace your hydrogenated oils with coconut oil. Or you could replace your store bought orange juice by eating fresh oranges.

Every small change helps. Once your diet is on point and you are on the IF plan, you will become a fat burning furnace. You will lose the fat much faster and also notice that you feel more energetic and overall, you feel better.

You will not be able to explain it. Your moods will get better. You will feel more lively and generally, life will seem much better. It may amaze you that the cloud that was hanging over you so long seems to have lifted.

That's the power of a clean diet.

CHAPTER 5 – A DAY IN THE LIFE OF IF

It would be extremely difficult to give an IF plan for you to follow because individuals have different needs and schedules. However, here are a few tips that you should adhere to when planning out your program.

Know your goals

If you are adopting the intermittent fasting plan to lose weight, you should know your calorie numbers. You should know how many calories to eat for you to be at a caloric deficit of about 500 calories daily.

If you're trying to build your body, you will have to be at a caloric surplus. So, you will need to consume all your calories within your eating window. This may actually be difficult if you're consuming a lot of calories. However, you will be less likely to gain fat.

If you are happy with your weight, then you can carry on eating whatever you're eating at the moment. It would be a good idea to check if your diet is healthy. All you need to do is fit all your meals within your eating window.

Know your schedule

Intermittent fasting is generally not focused on the foods you eat. It is focused on the timing. Your eating times and cut-off times are the cornerstones of intermittent fasting. You must comply with them for IF to be beneficial.

Many people who embark on IF usually find that their lives are controlled by their eating windows and fasting windows. They need to constantly check the timing and plan things out.

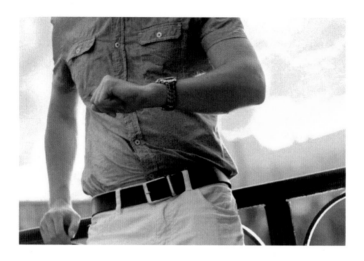

All these inconveniences can be avoided with proper planning.

Look at your schedule and preferences. What time do you wake up? What time is your lunch break at work? Do you prefer eating upon waking or would you rather go to sleep on a full stomach?

It is vital that you know your schedule and preferences. If you like going to bed with a full stomach, you'll probably have to schedule your eating window to start 6 hours after waking.

What if you're at work and get hungry? Will you be able to take a break to eat your first meal when your eating window opens?

All these are considerations you must bear in mind when planning your fasting.

How many meals will you eat?

Some people may prefer to eat throughout the eating window with several small meals. Other may opt for 1 or 2 big meals. Either way, it doesn't really matter... but you need to know which you prefer and plan it out.

When are you working out?

It is ideal that you embark on a regular exercise program. However, you need to know what time you will be training. Will you train on an empty stomach?

It's important to eat after a workout so that you body gets the fuel it needs and this will also boost your metabolic rate. So, plan your eating window in a manner where you're able to eat after you train.

CHAPTER 6 – COMMON INTERMITTENT FASTING MISTAKES TO AVOID

There are several mistakes that many people make when it comes to intermittent fasting. All of these mistakes can be avoided.

Mistake 1 – Giving up too fast

You must understand that intermittent fasting is the total opposite of what most people are accustomed to. All your life, you have not given much thought to eating times and ate whenever you've felt like it.

Adopting the IF method will be difficult initially. This is a given. You should mentally prepare yourself to stay the course for 2 weeks. Do not throw in the towel just because you slip up every now and then.

It is almost inevitable that you will slip up. You might get hungry and eat something. After this you will feel guilty and curse yourself for being weak. You might then decide that the entire plan has failed... and you quit.

This is the usual process that many newbies go through. Never quit. If you do slip up and eat something, keep your meal small.

The quest is not a failure if you keep at it.

Over time, your appetite will decrease and you will be more disciplined. It will become easier to stick with the plan. In fact, usually after 2 or 3 weeks, most people on IF find it more difficult to consume all their calories within the eating window.

From craving for food, they now feel like they have too much to eat and too little time. You will be amazed to see how fast your body adapts. Stick with the plan.

Mistake 2 – Poor planning

As mentioned earlier, timing is crucial with the intermittent fasting program. If you plan poorly, you will be stressing yourself out unnecessarily and constantly watching the clock. Intermittent fasting can be stressful in the beginning. You shouldn't add on to the stress with poor planning.

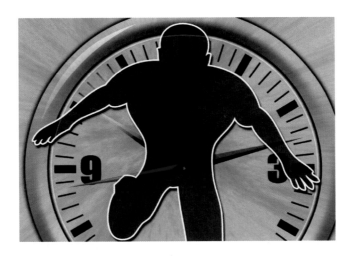

Mistake 3 – Being too ambitious

There are several different types of intermittent fasting. Many beginners want fast weight loss results. So, they adopt the fasting diet that involves 24 hour fasting or they cut their calories drastically and adopt IF.

Slow and steady wins the race. If you try to do too much too soon, the entire process will become torturous and stressful. It will just be a matter of time when your will-power will fail you and you will quit.

Start small and have a shorter fasting window. As the days progress, you can gradually increase the duration of your fasting window.

Mistake 4 – Not watching their diet

All calories are not made equal. Getting 400 calories from a piece of lean meat is different from getting 400 calories from 2 bars of chocolate.

Intermittent fasting does allow some leeway with your diet but if you want faster results with your fat loss, you should also eat a healthy and wholesome diet.

Your diet and IF are not mutually exclusive. You have everything to gain and nothing to lose by adopting a clean diet. Combine it with IF and you will burn the fat much faster.

Mistake 5 – Not exercising

Yes... it's hard work. Yes... you can lose weight with IF and a healthy diet. However, if you want to be stronger and fitter, you MUST exercise.

Ideally, you should have a mix of cardio and resistance training in your workouts. You can keep things interesting by trying varied workouts or even different types of exercises. Pilates on one day, kickboxing the next day or maybe swim some laps on the weekend.

The key is to move more and challenge yourself. Exercise is a habit. It is a difficult habit to inculcate but it's an extremely easy one to lose.

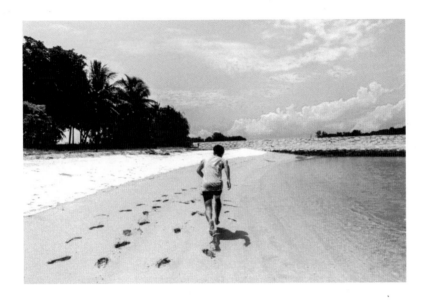

Intermittent fasting will help you lose weight and exercise will not only speed up the process but in the long run, it will keep off the fat. It is a fact that most people are able to lose weight but are often unable to keep the weight off for long.

The key to training is to build up your strength and stamina gradually. Have scheduled days to train and days to rest. NEVER skip a day of training because you're not in the mood.

Once you do this, you will find that you do not have the mood to exercise the next day too... and before you know it, you've stopped training for 3 weeks. Now, you need to struggle all over again to get the ball rolling.

If you don't want to lose momentum, don't stop for too long. Short 1 day rest days are sufficient. If you're not overtraining, 1 day of rest every 3 days is enough to give your body a break.

Now that you know what the common mistakes are, you can avoid them and attain success with intermittent fasting.

CHAPTER 7 – SHOULD I EXERCISE WHILE FASTING?

As mentioned earlier, yes... you definitely should.

There are many benefits of exercise such as:

- A higher metabolic rate which aids in fat loss
- It releases endorphins which will make you feel happier
- Prevents muscle atrophy. If you don't use it, you lose it.
- Improves blood circulation
- Prevents diseases that cause cognitive decline
- Encourages better sleep
- Keeps your weight under control
- And much, much more!

It may require Herculean effort to go from a sedentary lifestyle to an active one. The key here is small improvements daily. If you've not been exercising for years, you can start with a 20 minute walk daily.

Do not jump into a high intensity workout overnight. Give your body time to adapt and recover. Start with low impact exercises such as walking, cycling and swimming. Then move on to resistance training with light weights.

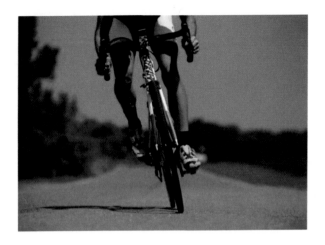

There is no need to train to the point of exhaustion when you're starting out. What matters is that you move more and get into the habit of exercising regularly. Over time, you can increase the intensity of your workouts and challenge yourself.

Do note that it is ok to train on an empty stomach but it is preferable that within 45 minutes from completion of your workout, you should have a meal. So, you could either train during your eating window or start your eating window after your workout.

That pretty much sums it up. A clean diet, intermittent fasting… and regular exercise are the three sides to the weight loss triangle. When you have all three components in place, you will lose weight, get healthier and fitter and keep the excess pounds off.

CONCLUSION

The intermittent fasting program is extremely effective, safe and sustainable. One of the biggest benefits of IF is that you could adopt it for life.

Unlike a fad diet which only works for a short while, intermittent fasting is a way of life. You will be eating real food and getting all the macronutrients you need. There are no restrictions.

The fasting window will take care of the fat burning process. Your body will also have more energy because it is not constantly digesting food. Your insulin levels will be more stable and your insulin sensitivity will improve.

This will make you less likely to gain weight.

If you're planning to adopt intermittent fasting, you absolutely should give it a try. Stay focused and committed. It will be difficult initially but nothing worth having ever came easy. As long as you stay the course, you will get accustomed to it and there will be no looking back.

Monitor your progress and how you feel. Write it all down in a journal. In a few weeks, you will see that you made an excellent decision by adopting intermittent fasting. Once you see the benefits, you can tell your friends and family about it and encourage them to join you.

"Instead of using medicine, rather, fast a day." - Plutarch.